CC

LIVING WITH DISEASE

CANCER

BY BILL McAULIFFE

CREATIVE EDUCATION

Contents

By the age of 25, Lance Armstrong

was already a world-champion bicycle racer. But his life changed when doctors found he had cancer of the **testicles** that had spread to his lungs and brain. A generation before, testicular cancer was fatal. Even Armstrong was given only a 50 percent chance of long-term survival. Armstrong had one testicle removed, underwent brain surgery, and endured months of rigorous treatment. Three years later, in 1999, he won the 2,200-mile (3,540 km) Tour de France and went on to become the first man to win the famous bicycle race seven years in a row. Armstrong has also become one of the world's most visible advocates for aggressiveness in fighting cancer, at both the community and the personal level. In 2009, at age 37, he came out of retirement and finished third in the Tour de France. "I'm racing for one reason," he said, "and that's to alleviate this disease around the world."

Lance Armstrong started the Lance Armstrong Foundation to advocate on behalf of cancer survivors in 1997.

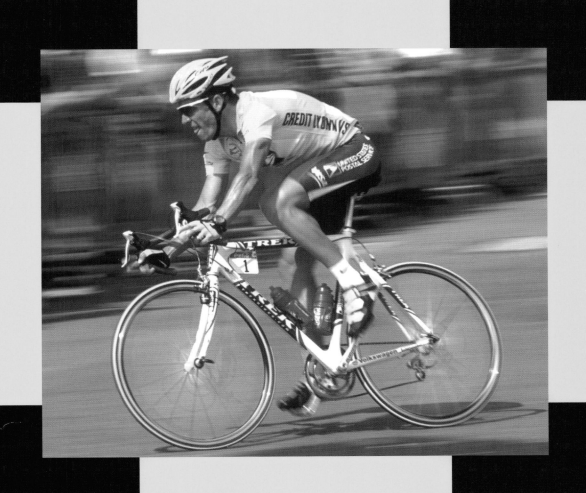

CHAPTER ONE

CANCEROUS FORMS

A cancer diagnosis is one of the

most dreaded things a patient can hear from a doctor. Most people regard the disease as a sort of monster against which they have no defense. Cancer can indeed be deadly, but as scientists have discovered more about it, they have been able to describe a threat with many dimensions—some of them severe and some of them less so.

A cancerous skin tumor (opposite) can be detected at the microscopic level.

Cancer is actually a group of more than 100 diseases with different origins, behaviors, and likely outcomes. Some cancers, such as cancer of the **pancreas**, are life-threatening. But many, such as skin cancers, are treatable. A century ago, fewer than 20 percent of people diagnosed with cancer survived. Today, almost 70 percent of cancer patients will be alive 5 years after their diagnosis.

One of every two men and one of every three women in the United States will get some sort of cancer in their lifetimes, but most will die of something else. Still, among all causes of death, cancer tops the list in Canada (at 25 percent) and comes in a close second to heart disease in the U.S. (at 23 percent). Worldwide, the cancer death rate is about half

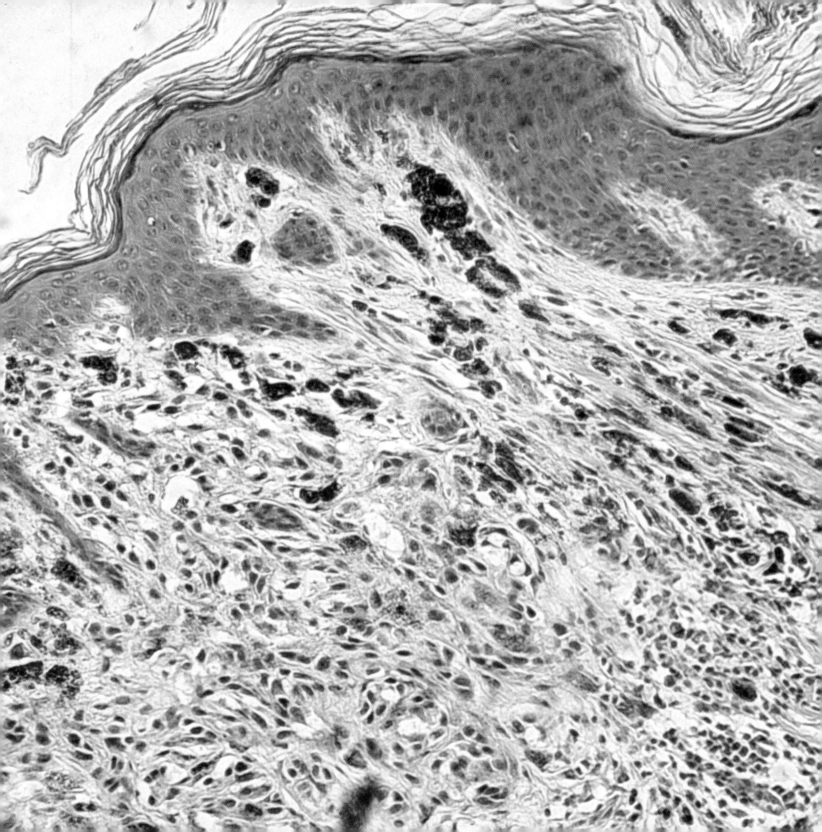

Cancer accounted for 13 percent (7.4 million) of all deaths globally in 2004. The most frequently fatal were cancer of the lung (1.3 million deaths), stomach (803,000), colon/rectum (639,000), liver (610,000), and breast (519,000). More than 70 percent of cancer deaths occurred in low- and middle-income countries.

that. That is because people in poorer countries die from heart disease, HIV/AIDS, and infectious diseases such as **tuberculosis** (TB) at higher rates than in wealthier nations.

Lung cancer claims the greatest share of cancer deaths in the U.S., followed by breast cancer for women and **prostate** cancer for men. In Canada, the top killers are lung and **colorectal** cancer. But the picture is not entirely grim. In the U.S., the cancer death rate and the rate at which people were diagnosed actually declined from 1975 to 2006, the latest year for which official figures were available. In Canada, rates for most major cancers have also been declining in recent years.

Physicians first recognized cancer more than 2,000 years ago, but it was present long before then. Scientists have found evidence of cancer in Ethiopian mummies from 3000 B.C. and even in dinosaur bones from millions of years ago. Around 400 B.C., the Greek physician Hippocrates named the disease. Because the swollen veins surrounding cancerous tumors looked like crab legs, Hippocrates applied the Greek name for "crab," *karkinos*, to the condition.

The Roman physician Galen, who lived from about A.D. 130 to 200, used the word *onkos*, Greek for "mass," to describe cancer. As a result, cancer specialists today are called oncologists. Hippocrates and Galen

The Hippocratic Oath historically taken by all doctors to practice medicine ethically was named after Hippocrates.

believed that cancer and all other diseases were caused by an imbalance of fluids, or "humors," in the body. This theory held firm for more than 1,400 years, until surgeons began performing **autopsies** regularly and learning more about the nature of disease.

While cancer has afflicted people throughout history, it was rarer in the past than it is now, simply because people didn't live long enough to develop advanced cases. They most often died from other diseases or accidents first, and women frequently died in childbirth. Today, many life-threatening cancers are diagnosed most commonly in people approaching 65 years of age.

Cancers can affect almost any part of the body and are usually named for the site at which they first form. Additionally, cancers are often categorized based on the more general types of body structures they colonize. Cancers of the skin or organ linings are called carcinomas. About 80 percent of cancers—including breast, intestinal, stomach, colon, lung, **vaginal**, and skin cancers—are carcinomas. Sarcomas are cancers of the connective tissues, such as bone, cartilage, muscle, or even fat. Lymphomas reside in the **lymphatic** system, glioma is in the brain, and leukemia refers to cancers of the blood or **bone marrow**.

Cancers do not always remain where they began; they can also metastasize, or spread to other parts of the body. Lung cancer frequently spreads to the brain, for example. Breast cancer often spreads to the lungs or bones. Because the liver functions as a filter, it is the organ where the most cancers spread and often receives cancers that originated in the colon, pancreas, and even the skin.

Although lung, prostate, breast, and colon cancer are the most common fatal cancers, skin cancer affects more people than any other type. Most skin cancers develop in the outer layer of the skin. They are treatable and rarely spread to other parts of the body. But a small proportion, called melanomas, which form in the cells that give people their skin color, are far more dangerous. They can spread through the body, and they lead to far more deaths than any other kind of skin cancer.

Cancers are often first detected by a lump, known as a tumor, which is made up of a mass of cancerous cells. Other outward signs of cancer include a sore that doesn't heal; a change in the size or appearance of a wart or mole; a cough that gets worse; weakness, weight loss, or exhaustion; or swelling of the lymph nodes, often described as "swollen glands." Sometimes blood tests will show evidence of cancer, too.

Father of the Pap Smear

Born in Greece, George Nicholas Papanicolaou earned his medical degree at the University of Athens in 1904. After serving in the military, he and his wife moved to the U.S., where he worked as a rug merchant, violinist, and clerk before being hired as a researcher at Cornell University. There, he studied vaginal cells from guinea pigs to learn more about cell changes during **menstrual** cycles. In translating what he learned to humans, Papanicolaou discovered that he could easily detect cancer or the potential for cancer in a woman's cervix by examining cells on a slide under a microscope. He publicized his findings in 1928, but it took more than two decades for his inexpensive method to be widely accepted as the best way to detect **cervical** cancer. The **Pap smear**, as it is now called, has led to a decrease of more than 70 percent in deaths from cervical cancer.

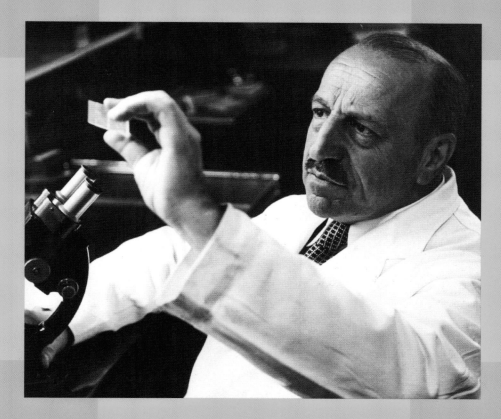

Dr. Papanicolaou worked at Cornell University in New York from 1913 until a few months before his 1962 death.

CANCEROUS FORMS

The physical signs of cancer are used to detect the disease in both adults and children. In the U.S., more than 10,000 children ages 14 and under are diagnosed with the disease annually. Of those, almost one-third are diagnosed with some form of leukemia, usually acute lymphocytic leukemia. This disease, in which too many white blood cells are formed in the blood, harms the body's ability to fight infections and also leads to bruising and unusual bleeding. Fortunately, about 80 percent of children with this disease are cancer-free 5 years after diagnosis and treatment. Most can expect that the disease will never return.

Brain cancer and cancers of other parts of the **nervous system** are the second-most common forms of childhood cancer. They make up about one in five childhood cancer cases. These cancers rarely spread to other parts of the body. About three out of four children with brain or nervous system cancers are cancer-free five years after diagnosis and treatment, although in some cases, the cancer can return.

The American Cancer Society calculates that the highest percentages of cancer deaths among men are from lung cancer (29 percent), prostate cancer (11 percent), and colorectal cancer (9 percent). For women's cancer deaths, the figures are 26 percent for lung cancer, 15 percent for breast cancer, and 9 percent for colorectal cancer.

CHAPTER TWO

MUTATION MECHANICS

Cancer is caused when cells

reproduce, or duplicate, uncontrollably. A healthy human body contains an estimated 100 trillion cells, which are the smallest structural units of any living organism. Different cells carry out different jobs in the body. Brain cells are responsible for thinking and operating the senses, muscles, and nerves. Red blood cells carry oxygen throughout the body, and white blood cells fight infection and destroy foreign substances. Cells in the pancreas help the body convert blood sugar into energy. Cells in a mother's breast produce milk for newborns.

The process of cell division for the majority of cells in the body is called mitosis.

Cell reproduction allows the body to grow and maintain itself. Cells receive signals instructing them to reproduce from substances within their own walls or from neighboring cells. They also get the instructions from **proteins** and sometimes from substances called growth factors, both of which flow within the bloodstream. When a cell gets a signal to reproduce, it makes an exact copy of all of its approximately 30,000 **genes** and splits into 2 identical cells. Each cell in a healthy human body reproduces about 60 times before it dies.

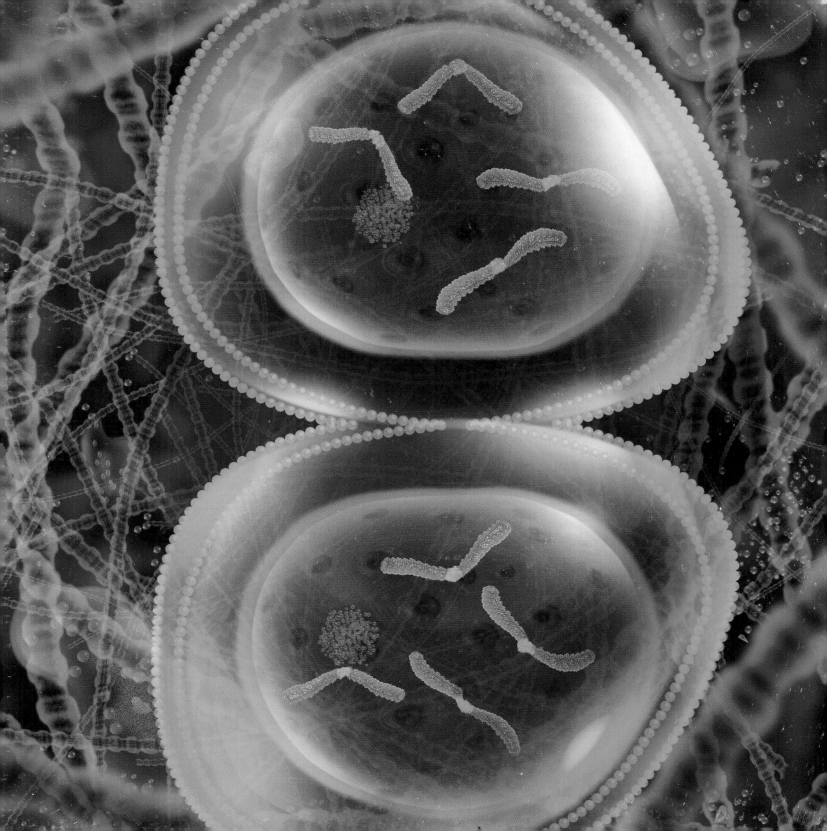

MUTATION MECHANICS

Cell division happens hundreds of millions of times a day in a person's body. And cells have their own mechanisms for making sure the process doesn't get out of control. Sometimes, though, a cell can have a defect in its genes, called a **mutation**, that causes the regulators to fail and allows tumors to form.

Healthy cells contain genes whose role is to limit cell duplication once it is underway. This normally stops the development of tumors, which means that a healthy body can prevent cancer all by itself. But if these regulatory genes become defective, cells can freely multiply and form tumors. A mutated gene can also cause a cell to act as though it's receiving orders for cell division when it isn't. The cell will then continue reproducing and won't die when it normally should; instead, cells will build up and form tumors. Mutant cells can multiply millions of times before they're detected as cancer.

Cancer cells can also break away from tumors and travel to other parts of the body through the bloodstream or lymphatic system. The migration of cancer cells from the point of origin to another body part is known as metastasis. Cancer cells are able to do this because they can sustain themselves by building their own blood vessels, which can carry

A New Focus on Genes

J. Michael Bishop grew up as a musician, and Harold Varmus earned a graduate degree in literature. But after following their passion for science, the two men wound up as research partners at the University of California, San Francisco. In 1975, while studying chickens, Bishop and Varmus proved that cancer was caused by gene mutations, not by an invasion from cells elsewhere in the body. That notion changed the basic understanding of cancer and led to an explosion of research into treatments targeted at genes. It also prompted Bishop to observe that "the seeds of cancer are within us." Bishop and Varmus's discovery showed that, while cancer can be inherited, it is most often spurred by environmental factors that can lead to gene mutations and often afflicts older people because mutations take time to multiply. The researchers, who were also close friends, shared the 1989 Nobel Prize in Physiology or Medicine.

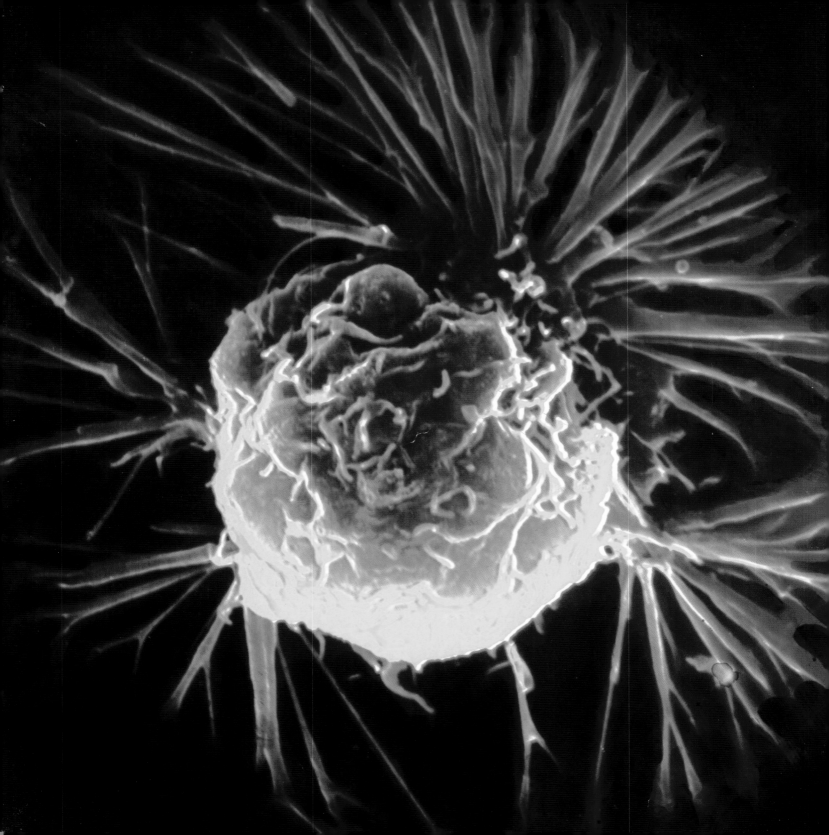

oxygen and other nutrients to the cells in a process called angiogenesis. Although they've changed location, the cancer cells are the same; lung cancer that has metastasized to the brain, for example, introduces cancerous lung cells into the brain. It is not called brain cancer but metastatic lung cancer.

In some patients, doctors find a metastatic cancer first. For example, prostate cancer, which sometimes shows few symptoms, might metastasize to a man's bones, causing lower back pain. This pain might be the first sign that anything is wrong. Doctors looking for the source of the back pain might find the prostate cancer cells in the bones and determine that the patient has a primary cancer in the prostate gland—something they would not have known to look for otherwise. Doctors are usually able to trace the origin of a metastasized cancer by the appearance of the cells; breast cancer cells, for example, look the same no matter where they've metastasized.

Because genes are often what trigger cancer, the disease is not contagious, like influenza or the measles. Some forms of cancer, such as breast, colon, or ovarian cancer, seem to take hold in certain families, as the gene is passed down from parent to child. But the majority of cancers come from a random gene mutation, not an inherited faulty gene.

The surface features of a breast cancer cell can be seen using a scanning electron microscope.

There are many ways genes can mutate and cause cancer. In modern society, people are often exposed to chemicals in the environment that can lead to genetic mutations and cancer. In 1775, a London physician named Percival Pott discovered that male chimney sweeps (people whose job was to clean the soot from dirty chimneys) had an unusually high incidence of cancer of the **scrotum**. Pott's finding was the first link between an occupation and a specific type of cancer.

The best-known cancer-causing substance in the environment is tobacco. Tobacco and tobacco smoke contain more than 60 chemicals known to cause cancer. In 1964, at a time when smoking was a popular and even glamorous habit, U.S. Surgeon General Luther Terry declared smoking an official public health threat. He reported that smokers were 9 to 10 times more likely to develop lung cancer than nonsmokers. In the 20th century, many workers exposed to asbestos, a mineral used to make fire-retardant and insulating products, developed a deadly form of cancer called mesothelioma. Unlike cancers that have many causes, mesothelioma is almost always linked to asbestos exposure.

Radiation can trigger many kinds of cancer by causing genes to mutate (although it can also cure the disease by killing cancerous cells). People have to be careful about how much radiation they're exposed to.

About 80 percent of lung cancer cases are attributed to smoking, according to the World Health Organization (WHO). Globally, tobacco kills 5.4 million people each year, and the WHO expects that figure to exceed 8 million by 2030. Lung cancer kills about 160,000 people in the U.S. every year.

According to the 1960–62 National Health and Nutrition Examination Survey, 13 percent of American adults ages 20 to 74 were obese. That number increased to 34 percent in 2010. Obesity may contribute to the occurrence of 25 to 30 percent of cancers such as colon and kidney cancer and breast cancer in older women.

CANCER

Hospital workers who conduct X-ray exams have to track their exposure to radiation. So do workers in nuclear power plants, where radiation leaks might occur. Naturally occurring radiation is also a cancer risk. Radon, which is emitted from soil, can build up in the basements of buildings and is the second-leading cause of lung cancer in the U.S. Even sunshine poses a cancer risk, as the **ultraviolet** (UV) radiation in sunlight can cause skin cancer.

Skin cancer and lung cancer have something in common that other cancers do not: they can both be avoided—lung cancer by not smoking, and skin cancer by using sunscreen and limiting one's exposure to the sun. **Obesity**, often a result of a lack of exercise and a poor diet, is another lifestyle link to cancer, particularly colon, kidney, and breast cancer. Dr. Otis Brawley, chief medical officer for the American Cancer Society, called obesity "the second-largest carcinogen" in the U.S., trailing only smoking as a cancer risk factor.

People are advised to wear sunscreen year round to protect themselves from harmful UV rays.

CHAPTER THREE

CONFRONTING CANCER

Because cancer is a disease with so many different forms, there are many different ways to treat it. Some cancers, such as prostate cancer or certain forms of leukemia, are slow to develop and may not even require treatment before patients die of something else, often because they are aging and likely to develop other health problems. Other cancers, such as breast cancer, have the potential to expand rapidly and spread to other organs, thus requiring a quick and aggressive response.

Cancer can be detected in many ways. Some of the more common cancers are found through periodic tests designed specifically to find them, such as Pap smears for cervical and other related cancers or a type of X-ray known as a mammogram for breast cancer. Others, such as prostate cancer and leukemia, are found through blood tests.

Unseen tumors might press against nerves or organs, creating puzzling symptoms that send a patient to the doctor. A brain tumor, for example, might cause dizziness, speech problems, or headaches. Several scanning procedures can find hidden tumors. These include computer-

A person born in the U.S. today can expect to live 78 years. Children who died of cancer in 2006 lost an average of 71 years of that expected life. Lung cancer cost victims a total of 2,378,000 years of expected life, and breast cancer was second-costliest: 773,500 years.

ized tomography (CT) scans, which involve a series of rotating X-rays; magnetic resonance imaging (MRI), which uses radio waves and magnetic fields to detect energy signals being emitted by **atoms** in body tissues; positron emission tomography (PET) scans to measure emissions given off by injected **radioactive** material; and ultrasonography, which uses sound waves bounced off internal body structures.

Once a tumor has been detected, a doctor needs to determine whether it is cancerous or benign (non-cancerous). This is usually done with a biopsy, in which the doctor takes a small sample of the tumor's cells—often by scraping some away or withdrawing them through a needle—and examines them under a microscope. Cells that are irregularly shaped, varying in size, or disorderly in arrangement are key indicators of cancer.

If a tumor is benign, the doctor might leave it alone. But if it's cancerous, the doctor must evaluate the disease. Some cancers are called indolent, meaning they do not expand quickly. Oncologists often don't prescribe any specific treatment for these types of cancers unless symptoms such as pain, infections, bone loss, or bleeding begin to appear.

After examining sample cells of a tumor and its surroundings, doctors will often assign a "stage" to the cancer to describe the level of

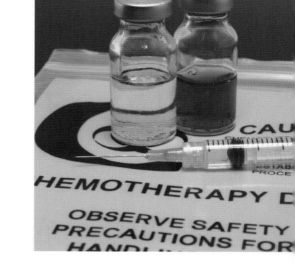

threat it poses and determine an appropriate treatment. Stages are assigned numbers (0, I, II, III, IV) to indicate the severity of the disease. At stage 0, a cancer is still in the cell layer where it started. At stage IV, it has metastasized and should receive immediate treatment.

The standard treatments for a fast-growing cancer include surgery, chemotherapy, and radiation, with most patients undergoing all three. Surgery has been the primary weapon used to fight cancer since the 1500s. Its aim is to remove the tumor and any cancerous tissue that surrounds it, including removing a diseased organ, or part of it, if necessary.

Chemotherapy, or the use of powerful drugs to destroy cells, has been employed in cancer therapy since the 1950s. Usually, chemotherapy drugs are given as a pill or in a solution injected directly into a vein every few weeks over the course of four to six months. The drugs are designed to attack cells in specific locations. Sometimes chemotherapy is used to shrink a tumor so that it can later be removed surgically. While killing cancer cells, chemotherapy also kills healthy cells. Because of this, chemotherapy often produces a side effect that has become symbolic of cancer: hair loss. Chemotherapy is not effective against some cancers, including cancers of the kidney, pancreas, and skin.

Chemotherapy drugs are cytotoxic, meaning they damage cells.

An Unforgettable Voice

Nat King Cole was one of the most popular performers in the U.S. in the 1940s and '50s. Although he first made his mark as a jazz pianist and bandleader, his career took off when he was featured as a singer. With a sophisticated style and a smooth, versatile voice, Cole recorded a number of hits, appeared in movies, and even had his own network television show. But Cole's success and his death were intertwined. Cole smoked three packs of cigarettes a day for much of his adult life. He insisted on smoking several cigarettes before performing because he said it added a husky quality to his voice. Cole died of lung cancer in 1965 at the age of 45. One of his best-known songs, "Unforgettable," was re-recorded by his daughter Natalie in 1991 as a duet, using Cole's voice 26 years after he had died.

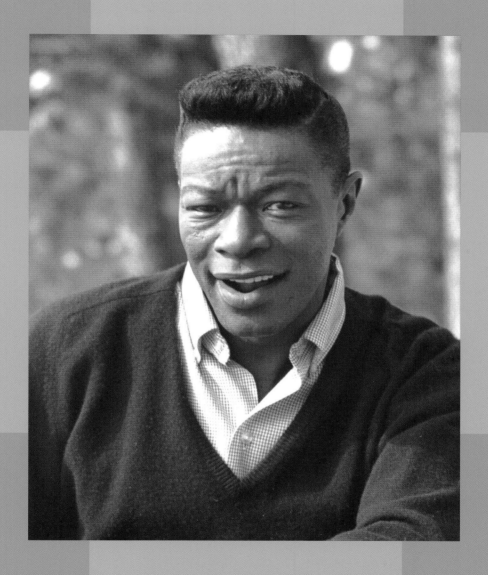

Nat King Cole, pictured in 1964, a year before his death from lung cancer.

The field of image-guided radiation therapy saw many improvements in the 1950s.

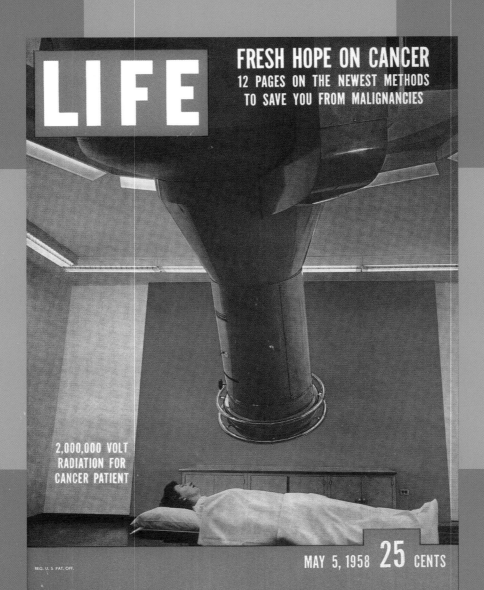

LIFE

FRESH HOPE ON CANCER
12 PAGES ON THE NEWEST METHODS
TO SAVE YOU FROM MALIGNANCIES

2,000,000 VOLT
RADIATION FOR
CANCER PATIENT

REG. U. S. PAT. OFF.

MAY 5, 1958 **25** CENTS

For more than a century, radiation therapy has been used to treat cancer. But the treatment came about at some cost to early researchers. In order to determine the proper amount of radiation for their patients, doctors would commonly test a radiation dose on their arms. They were trying to cause a pink spot to appear, which would indicate a correct dose. But many of these doctors were later diagnosed with leukemia, likely generated by gene mutations caused by the excessive exposure to radiation.

Radiation therapy is employed to combat nearly all types of cancer. Sometimes it's used as an alternative to surgery, since it can destroy a tumor by focusing energy many times more powerful than X-rays on the target. It can also be used to shrink or eliminate benign tumors. Like chemotherapy, radiation also kills healthy cells, but because it can be targeted, the damage can be limited. Researchers are investigating new drugs that might be given to patients to make radiation even more effective.

Radiation treatments are given in a hospital or clinic but usually require only a series of brief visits over weeks or months. They are also used to kill cancer cells that may have survived after tumors have been removed surgically or have disappeared through treatment. Radiation

The 5-year survival rate (the percentage of people still alive 5 years after their cancer diagnosis) for all races and ages of men diagnosed with prostate cancer leapt from 69 percent in 1975 to 99 percent in 2006. But the survival rate for people with pancreatic cancer was only 22.5 percent in 2006.

has its own side effects, including fatigue, sensitive skin, and mouth infections, as well as potential complications in the workings of the organ being treated.

Treatment doesn't always cure cancer. Survival rates vary widely for different cancers and treatments. In the face of advanced-stage cancers, doctors might still use surgery, chemotherapy, or radiation but only to reduce symptoms or postpone a patient's likely death. This is called palliative care. Meanwhile, cancer patients often consider using herbs, vitamins, and dietary changes to fight cancer. Other alternatives are massage, acupuncture (a method of inserting needles into the skin and nerves to cure disorders and reduce pain), and meditation, which uses quiet reflection and mental relaxation to relieve pain and stress. Many of these treatments are often recommended by doctors. The National Cancer Institute regards them as additions to—but not substitutes for— conventional treatments. The institute also warns that some alternatives may actually interfere with conventional methods by counteracting some of the beneficial effects of chemotherapy or drugs, or by leading a patient to postpone conventional therapy. The institute urges patients to carefully study such treatments—and the sources of information about them—before adopting the methods.

CHAPTER FOUR

SEARCHING FOR CURES

Although cancer has plagued humankind for centuries, research into its causes and possible treatments has progressed slowly. Physicians in the 19th century knew that what they called "true" tumors were made up of cells that had multiplied out of control. But in 1900, cancer was still only eighth on the list of causes of death in the U.S., far behind pneumonia, TB, and intestinal disorders. It wasn't until after World War II (1939–45), when cancer became one of the top two causes of death, that research began to accelerate. In 1971, U.S. president Richard Nixon signed the National Cancer Act, committing $100 million to cancer research. "The time has come in America when the same kind of concentrated effort that split the atom and took man to the moon should be turned toward conquering this dread disease," Nixon said.

Forty years later, researchers have developed treatments that have increased survival rates for many cancers. They've gained great understanding into how cancer works and how it might be thwarted. But they have also revealed just how diverse cancer is, how minute are its triggers, and how elusive its cures. Though the number of cancer cases and

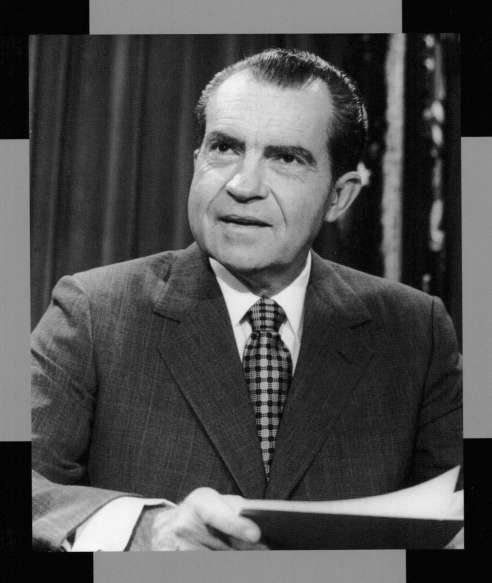

President Nixon first proposed funding cancer research in a January 1971 speech; the act was signed into law on December 23.

BY THE NUMBERS The U.S. states with the highest incidence rates of breast cancer from 2002 to 2006 were on opposite coasts. They included five eastern states—Connecticut (with 135 cases per 100,000 people), Massachusetts (132), New Hampshire (131), Vermont (130), and Maine (129)—plus Washington (135) and Oregon (132).

deaths has been declining in the U.S. and Canada, survival rates are still low for some kinds of cancer, particularly pancreas, liver, lung, and stomach cancers.

In the years following Nixon's initiative, research was characterized by a random search for chemicals that would kill cancer cells but not the patient. In 1975, researchers at the University of California, San Francisco discovered that cancer in chickens could be traced to a defective gene. Three years later, a researcher at the National Cancer Institute found a cancer-causing gene in rats that soon was also detected in 30 percent of human cancers, including 90 percent of pancreatic cancers and 50 percent of colon cancers. Those findings changed the nature of the battle against cancer, leading researchers to search for drugs that could disrupt the defective genes that cause the disease. This method of attacking cancer cells is called targeted therapy.

Unlike chemotherapy and radiation, which attack rapidly dividing cells regardless of whether they are cancerous or healthy, targeted therapy can spare healthy cells. But targeted therapy is often used along with chemotherapy and radiation because it can increase their effectiveness. One form of targeted therapy blocks **enzymes** from communicating growth signals to cancer cells, limiting their multiplication. Another alters proteins to cause cell death, a normal process that sometimes gets overridden. And because cancer cells can essentially cultivate their own blood vessels to give them nourishment, still another type of targeted therapy is designed to short-circuit this ability.

Two of the best-known targeted therapy drugs have been in widespread use for less than a decade. Imatinib mesylate attacks abnormal proteins that spark unlimited growth in certain cells and is used most often against cancers of the gastrointestinal tract and chronic myelogenous leukemia. Trastuzumab was developed to bind to and interfere with a protein that is common in 20 to 30 percent of breast cancers, particularly in those that are most aggressive. The protein, when defective, creates multiple receptors for growth signals, leading to rampant reproduction, so trastuzumab blocks the receptors. Targeted therapies are now being used against some types of lung, kidney, and bone marrow cancers as well.

Targeted therapies are not the miracle cure for cancer. Although these drugs have been successful in treating some cancers, others, such as leukemia, become **resistant** to the genetic tampering in which the drugs engage. In some cases, researchers have simply moved the target, finding another protein involved in cell reproduction to attack after

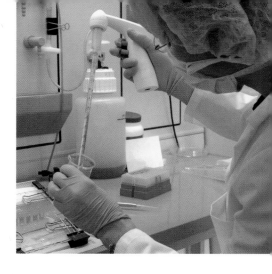

the first one resists the drug. But targeted therapies are expensive, and their effectiveness varies from patient to patient. So far, they've been used only in advanced cases of cancer.

Scientists are also researching **vaccines** that might help prevent the development of cancer in the first place. Already on the market is a vaccine that fights a sexually transmitted disease called human papillomavirus (HPV), which has been linked to cervical and other cancers in women. The vaccine wards off HPV, not the cancer, and it has to be taken before a woman becomes sexually active. Another available vaccine prevents a type of liver infection that can lead to cancer. In April 2010, the U.S. Food and Drug Administration approved a vaccine that would treat prostate cancer by stimulating the immune system's response to fighting tumors.

In addition to drugs and vaccines, researchers believe that gene therapy may hold some promise for derailing or even preventing cancer. Using gene therapy, scientists could add healthy genes to cells that have abnormal or missing genes or restore genes that help cells repair themselves. They could also change genes to make them more sensitive to chemotherapy and radiation or get them to work better with the body's

Scientists at many cancer research centers collaborate with other laboratories to find the best new therapies.

Cancer Quells the Lion

For decades, U.S. senator Edward "Ted" Kennedy had fought for putting better health care within reach of more Americans. But in the final year of his life, Kennedy's own health became a national story. The youngest brother of former president John F. Kennedy, Ted became 1 of only 6 people in U.S. history to serve more than 40 years (1962–2009) in the Senate. During his career, the "Lion of the Senate" helped pass major bills, such as those regarding children's health insurance, AIDS research, and the Family and Medical Leave Act. Kennedy was diagnosed with brain cancer in 2008, but he returned to the Senate to lead an effort to reform health insurance. "I've benefited from the best of medicine," he said, and thought that others should be entitled to the same. His vote on a Medicare bill was one of his final acts in the Senate. He died in August 2009.

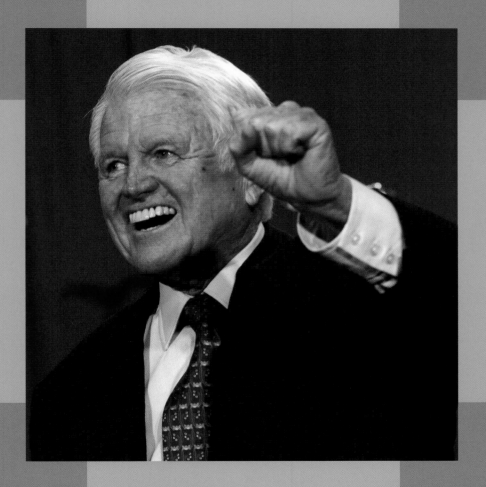

Senator Kennedy's
cancer treatments left
him prone to seizures,
but he continued his
work throughout
early 2009.

own immune system, which fights disease. Gene therapy was used successfully for the first time in 2006, when the immune system cells of 15 melanoma patients were injected with genes that enabled them to attack cancer cells. In two of the patients, the new genes mobilized the body's own immune system to fight their cancerous tumors, which were wiped out within a year.

Drugs and technology remain at the center of cancer research, but prevention is also being emphasized. With some studies showing that up to 90 percent of colorectal cancers might be connected to diets that are low in fiber and high in fat, experts now urge people to adhere to a healthy diet and to exercise as a way to reduce their risk of developing this type of cancer.

In the thousands of years since cancer was first recognized, scientists have come a long way in advancing their knowledge of the disease, and hope grows that many cancers may one day be cured. But cancer is a multidimensional disease, and much more remains to be learned before it can be conquered. Fortunately, although more people than ever have cancer, researchers are helping more people than ever survive it.

In the U.S., African American men have the highest cancer diagnosis rate (652 per 100,000 people) of any racial group, and Asian American women have the lowest (288). African American men also have the highest death rate (313) from cancer, while American Indian women have the lowest (95.6).

GLOSSARY

atoms: the smallest particles of an element that can exist alone

autopsies: examinations of a body's vital organs after death to determine the cause of death

bone marrow: the tissue within bones where blood cells are created

cervical: relating to the narrow passage that leads from a woman's uterus to the vagina (the canal that leads to the outside of the body)

colorectal: having to do with the last part of the large intestine, known as the colon, and the rectum, to which it leads

enzymes: proteins that trigger chemical reactions in the body

genes: the basic units of instruction in a cell, which control a person's physical traits and pass characteristics from parents to offspring

lymphatic: relating to lymph, a clear fluid containing white blood cells that travels through the body, carrying nutrients to cells and helping remove bacteria and prevent infection

menstrual: having to do with the monthly discharge of blood and tissue from the uterus in non-pregnant females

mutation: a change in genetic material that is relatively permanent, resulting in a new characteristic or function in a cell

nervous system: a network in the body that includes the brain and the spinal cord; it determines responses to sensations and controls basic bodily functions such as the heartbeat

obesity: the condition of having a body mass index greater than 30, which is a measurement of one's weight in relation to height

pancreas: a large gland near the intestines that aids in digestion and produces insulin

Pap smears: tests involving chemical coloring of cells to determine the presence of cervical cancer

prostate: a male gland that plays a role in sperm distribution

proteins: complex structures that are the basic components of all living cells

radiation: energy emitted by one body that can penetrate another

radioactive: relating to the spontaneous emission of energetic particles (such as electrons) as an atom decays

resistant: unaffected by the harmful effects of something, such as a drug

scrotum: the sac in most male mammals that contains the testicles

testicles: the male reproductive glands, which produce sperm

tuberculosis: an infectious disease that usually affects the lungs

ultraviolet: a form of radiation that comes from beyond the visible violet end of the light spectrum

vaccines: substances given in a shot or by mouth that help the immune system form antibodies (disease-fighting proteins) to fight off a specific disease

vaginal: having to do with the canal that leads from a woman's cervix (the passage below the uterus) to the outside of the body

BIBLIOGRAPHY

American Cancer Society. "Information and Resources for Cancer." American Cancer Society. http://www.cancer.org.

Canadian Cancer Society. "Home." Canadian Cancer Society. http://www.cancer.ca.

Coleman, C. Norman. *Understanding Cancer: A Patient's Guide to Diagnosis, Prognosis, and Treatment.* 2nd ed. Baltimore: Johns Hopkins University Press, 2006.

Gabriel, Janice. *The Biology of Cancer.* 2nd ed. Hoboken, N.J.: John Wiley & Sons, 2007.

Rather, L. J. *The Genesis of Cancer: A Study in the History of Ideas.* Baltimore: Johns Hopkins University Press, 1978.

U.S. National Institutes of Health. "Comprehensive Cancer Information." National Cancer Institute. http://www.cancer.gov.

Yount, Lisa, ed. *Cancer.* San Diego: Greenhaven Press, 2000.

FURTHER READING

Cefrey, Holly. *Coping with Cancer.* New York: Rosen Publishing Group, 2004.

Gold, John Coopersmith. *Cancer.* Berkeley Heights, N.J.: Enslow, 2001.

Massari, Francesca. *Everything You Need to Know about Cancer.* New York: Rosen Publishing Group, 2000.

Stoyles, Pennie. *The A–Z of Health.* Vol. 2, *C–E.* North Mankato, Minn.: Smart Apple Media, 2011.

INDEX

Published by Creative Education • P.O. Box 227, Mankato, Minnesota 56002
Creative Education is an imprint of The Creative Company
www.thecreativecompany.us
Design and production by The Design Lab • Art direction by Rita Marshall
Printed by Corporate Graphics in the United States of America
Photographs by Alamy (Editorial, Medicalpicture, Phototake Inc., www.geraldbrown.co.uk),
Corbis (Bettmann, Frank Lane Picture Agency, Jason Reed/Reuters), Getty Images (Esther Bubley/
Time & Life Pictures, Hulton Archive, Michael Ochs Archives), iStockphoto (Khuong Hoang, Dr.
Heinz Linke, Kyu Oh)

Library of Congress Cataloging-in-Publication Data
McAuliffe, Bill. Cancer / by Bill McAuliffe. p. cm. — (living with disease)
Includes bibliographical references and index. Summary: A look at cancer, examining the ways in
which the disease develops, its different forms and symptoms, the effects it has on a person's daily
life, and ongoing efforts to find a cure.
ISBN 978-1-60818-073-8
1. Cancer—Juvenile literature. I. Title. II. Series.
RC264.M33 2011   616.99'4—dc22   2010030363

CPSIA: 110310 PO1384
First Edition 9 8 7 6 5 4 3 2 1